Living with Aromatherapy and Essential Oil

How Aromatherapy and Essential Oils Enhance Your Emotional and Physical Wellbeing

By: Margaret J. Bilkins

9781681279596

Publishers Notes

Disclaimer – Speedy Publishing LLC

This publication is intended to provide helpful and informative material. It is not intended to diagnose, treat, cure, or prevent any health problem or condition, nor is intended to replace the advice of a physician. No action should be taken solely on the contents of this book. Always consult your physician or qualified health-care professional on any matters regarding your health and before adopting any suggestions in this book or drawing inferences from it.

The author and publisher specifically disclaim all responsibility for any liability, loss or risk, personal or otherwise, which is incurred as a consequence, directly or indirectly, from the use or application of any contents of this book.

Any and all product names referenced within this book are the trademarks of their respective owners. None of these owners have sponsored, authorized, endorsed, or approved this book.

Always read all information provided by the manufacturers' product labels before using their products. The author and publisher are not responsible for claims made by manufacturers.

This book was originally printed before 2015. This is an adapted reprint by Speedy Publishing LLC with newly updated content designed to help readers with much more accurate and timely information and data.

Speedy Publishing LLC

40 E Main Street, Newark, Delaware, 19711

Contact Us: 1-888-248-4521

Website: http://www.speedypublishing.co

REPRINTED Paperback Edition: 9781681279596

Manufactured in the United States of America

Dedication

I dedicate this book to my best friend Bridget. I would like to thank you for your support and encouragement.

Table of Contents

CHAPTER 1- A BRIEF HISTORY OF AROMATHERAPY

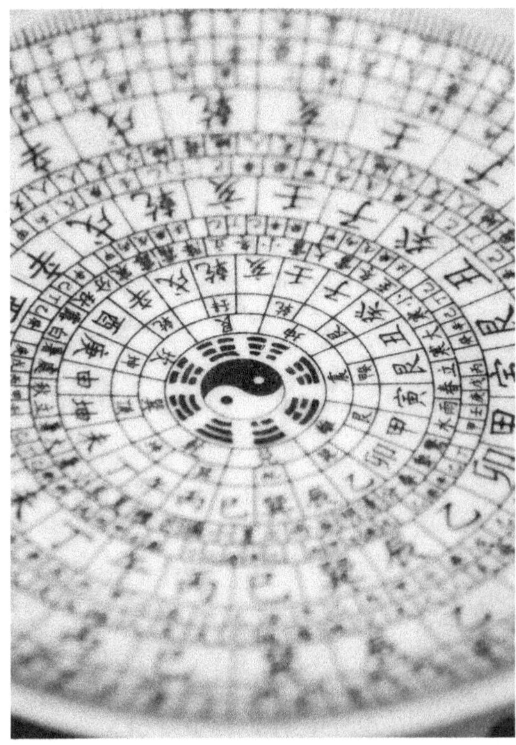

You have probably heard the term Aromatherapy and wondered what exactly that funny word, „aromatherapy" actually means. It is the use of plant oils in their most essential form to promote both mental and physical well being. The use of the word aroma implies the process of inhaling the scents from these oils into your lungs for therapeutic benefit.

The term aromatherapy is generally new, beginning to be used in the 20th century, but the practice has been around for thousands of years. It is believed that the Chinese were one of the first cultures to use the scents of plants to promote health through the burning of incense. Ancient Egyptians used distilled cedar wood oil mixed with clove, cinnamon, nutmeg, and myrrh to embalm the deceased. The Egyptians also used oils to perfume both men and women.

In the 14th century when the bubonic plague hit, killing thousands of people, aromas were used to ward off the deadly disease. There is even discussion that the popular nursery rhyme, "Ring around the Roses" refers to aromatherapy. The lines, "a pocket full of posies" allegedly refers to keeping the flower in ones pocket in an attempt to keep the illness away.

Moving forward through later centuries a growth in books about the use of oils in healing grew.

The Greek alchemist, Paracelsus, used the term "essence" and focused study on the use of plants for healing purposes.

While the use of essential oils for perfume continued to grow throughout the ages its" use for medicinal purposes waned slightly until around 1928.

It was at that time that a French chemist named Rene-Maurice Gattefosse accidentally discovered the use of lavender essential oil to heal wounds.

The story is told that he burned his forearm and reflexively placed it in the closest liquid he saw, which was lavender essential oil. He was surprised to find that the burn healed rapidly and left no scar. It was then that he began using the term aromatherapy and wrote about the powers of essential oils.

Today, many people are trying to get back to nature. People have seen firsthand the dangerous effects of synthetic chemicals and processed medications.

The use of all natural essential oils for medicinal, cosmetic and therapy purposes continues to grow. Many people have found the results of using aromatherapy to be far greater than manmade medications and with far fewer negative side effects.

Aromatherapy can be used by itself or in conjunction with typical medical treatments. For example, you may use aromatherapy to ease pain after a surgical procedure. You still get the benefit of the surgery but do not have to take the powerful and often dangerous pain medications that a doctor prescribes.

Chapter 2- The Basics of Aromatherapy & Essential Oils

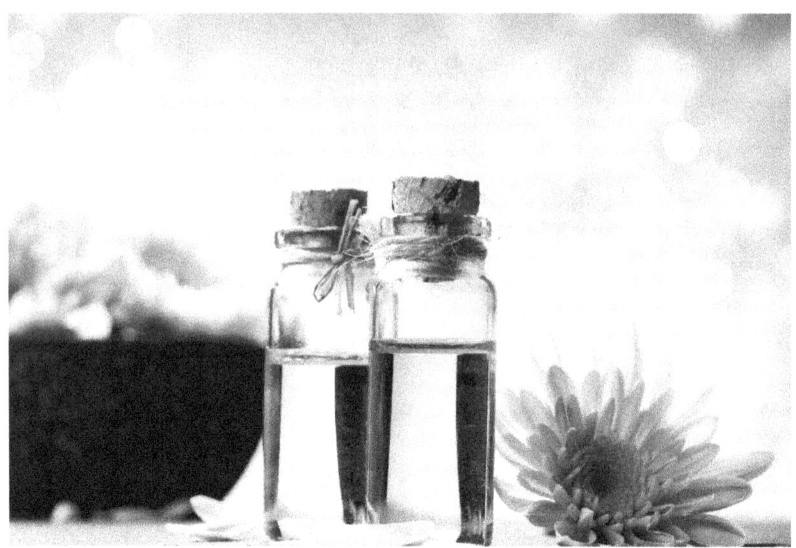

The importance of understanding a particular topic, idea, or element is often overlooked in this busy world of today. To make matters worse it is often difficult to find the time to really extensively explore particular topics. However with the use of various modern tools, this task can be not only fun but very informative too.

Most people today understand aromatherapy as just another indulgent exercise the privileged few enjoy. However upon taking the time to delve deeper, one is likely to find a whole new prospect relating to the very diverse uses of aromatherapy.

Aromatherapy can be explored as an alternative to more invasive methods of treatments. Originating long before medical science made discoveries and break-through; aromatherapy has had many success stories to back its many wondrous attributes. The concept of using aromatherapy to treat wounds and burns first came about when a scientist badly burned his hand while conducting an experiment and later it was used again successfully, as an antiseptic to treat the wounded soldiers during world war two.

Being the basis of natural materials, aromatherapy is less dangerous a method to choose from, when deciding on the best suited treatment for various illnesses. In theory aromatherapy is a treatment that may or may not help in the prevention of diseases by the use of essential oils. When coupled with the more conventional methods of treatments it has been found to produce impressive results, mainly contributing as a calming ingredient to the equation.

Aromatherapy can have a positive impact on the limbic system through the olfactory system. It has also been known to have direct pharmacologic effects. There have been studies done to prove the connection between the direct impacts of use between aromatherapy coupled with other scientific methods, however to date no conclusive data has been forth coming.

Aromatherapy works to heal the mind and body. The natural herbs, oils, fragrances, etc aid in healing a wide array of diseases. At most aromatherapy reduces irritating symptoms, as well as emotional negativity's. Aromatherapy is used to heal the mind by relieving stress.

Down through the century's aromatherapy has been used by a wide selection of professionals and individuals alike. India natives, Egyptians, Germans, Frenchmen, Europeans, Brazilians, etc, have all used and still use aromatherapy oils. After ongoing studies, research, etc, the oils has proven to assist in promoting health. In fact, medical doctors use aromatherapy in medical treatment. On the market is a variety of aromatherapy scented and essential oils. The oils include Asafoetida, Cajuput, Celery Seed, Jasmine, Black Currant Seed, Carrot Seed, Bergamot, Basil, and so on. Absinthe, Ajowan, African Bluegrass, Anise Star, Anethi, Australian Balm Mint

Bush, Arborvitae Wild are a variety of other oils available on the market.

Australian Balm Latin name is Prostandthera Melissifolia. The flowery plant was extracted through steam process. The oils origin is Australia, which its flowers is shaped similar to a purple bell. The oils are pale yellow once extracted, and works as an anti-bacterial agent. The oils work as anti-fungal agents as well. Australian Balm will help reduce colic, headaches, and colds. The medium scented oil blends with peppermint, lavender, lemongrass, spearmint, and citronella. The oils are non-toxic and are used as a cooking ingredient as well.

Ajowan is an essential oil, which its Latin name is Trachyspermum Copticum. The herbs were extracted through a steam distillation process. The origin of ajowan starts in India. Ajowan produces pale, yellowish brown oils. The oils are essential for stimulating, and are used as anti-spasmodic agents. In addition, ajowan has microbial agents, and properties that help to fight colic symptoms. The strong scent blends with sage, thyme, and parsley.

Ajowan is sometimes called Bishop Weed. The oils originated in India, yet they are widely used in Egypt, Iran, Afghanistan, and Pakistan. You must dilute the oils before applying to the skin, otherwise it could cause irritation. If you're pregnant it is recommended that you do not use the oils.

Anise Star in Latin is called Illicium Verum. The oils are extracted through steam distillation process, and come from plant seeds. In addition, Anise Star originates in China, yet it has a well-known usage in various lands. Anise is a plant that grows licorice flavored seeds. The Mediterranean plants are used in medicines, and to flavor drink and foods. The Latin name is Pimpinella Anisum. The oils are clear, or light yellow. Moreover, the oils are used to treat colic, rheumatism, and are used in cough syrups, as well as pastille.

The light scented oils blend with orange, lavender, pine, clove, cinnamon, and rosewood. The oil is used in various lands as well as a breath freshener and aid to clear up the digestive system.

Arborvitae Wild is an essential oil, which its botanic name is Thuja OCCIDENTALIS. The extraction of the needle and twigs from plants occurred through a steam distillation process. The origin of these plants is Canada. Arborvitae Wild is a confer tree, which is akin to the cypress family. The flat leaves fit closely, which the leaves resemble scales.

The oils are pale yellow, which the oil is used as an anti-rheumatic agent, anti-infection solution, anti-allergenic aid, etc. The oil is also used as an insect repellent. In addition, you can use this oil as an anti-inflammatory agent, to treat poison ivy, as an anti-microbial agent, etc. The strong scented oils blend with cinnamon Bark, birch sweet, eucalyptus, Cedarwood, cajuput, and cassia oils. Arborvitae Wild is considered the oils of from the trees of life. The oils were used to ward off lightning. Arborvitae Wild oils are to be used as instructed. We can now learn how to use aromatherapy.

Chapter 3- What Everyone Should Know About Aromatherapy

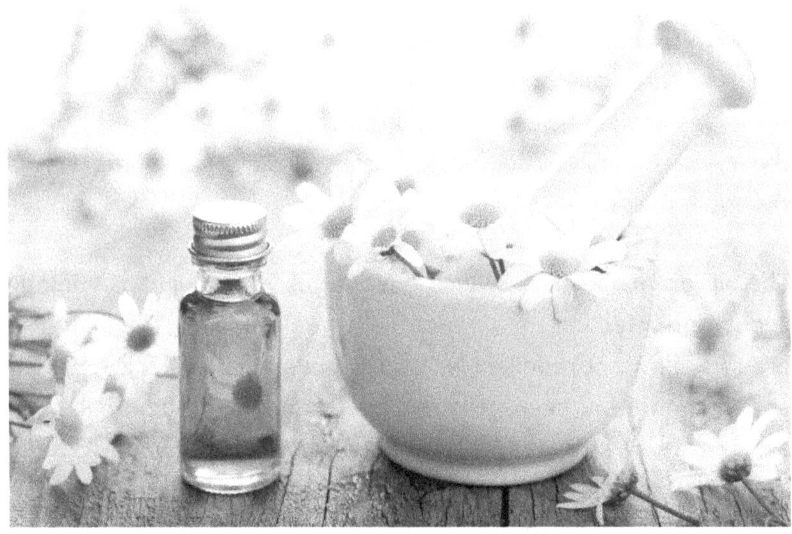

Some consider aromatherapy as a new age alternative style of treatment, while yet others know of its origins that date back a long while.

Indulging in aromatherapy is a choice that should only be made after understanding the various aspects of this field. This is most important when choosing aromatherapy as an alternative to medical treatments when trying to arrest, cure or prevent diseases.

The general perception of aromatherapy is, getting the scent of an essential oil to infuse itself into the atmosphere to create a pleasing and relaxing state of body and mind. To others is may be perceived as a relaxing massage session with the use of beneficial essential oils.

Using aromatherapy as a skin care regimen is also very popular. Many of the essential oils used have proven qualities that can contribute to the various needs addressed in skin care lines.

These requirements can range from wanting to keep the skin looking young and supple to actually reversing the aging effects on the skin. Some forms of eczema and acne have been successfully arrested with the use of the aromatherapy method.

Aromatherapy is also an excellent way recommended to get oneself into a meditative state. These meditative states are usually associated with yoga, tai chi, visualization or self hypnosis.

Trying various oils before deciding on the one that best allows you to reach the required level of mediation is sometimes needed. Besides this some research has shown that using aromatherapy can help create the mood for various scenarios with specific results in mind.

Though there is lack of conclusive evidence to show aromatherapy can be instrumental in treating certain diseases, the fact remains that many people turn to this alternative based on other success stories.

Traditionally linked to the successful treatment of emotional and physical ailments there is proven success because aromatherapy is a natural method that helps the body cope with stress, anxiety and tension which are all contributing factors or causes of other illnesses and diseases.

Aromatherapy has become very popular today. Though it is still mostly linked to idea of a relaxingly therapeutic massage session, newer uses are now being explored.

In ancient times aromatherapy was used for almost everything from relaxing to health solutions and even for culinary preparations. A lot needs to be understood before embarking on the journey of aromatherapy.

If one is thinking of setting up an aromatherapy centre or even considering the use of aromatherapy to treat a certain medical condition, the buying of the essential oils is a crucial aspect to consider.

Most essential oils today are so commercialized that it may not always be as genuine as stated on the labels. Careful examination of the label contents needs to be checked and rechecked before a purchase is made.

Some labels can be quite deceiving in their purported capabilities. The condition and type of packing of the essential oils is also a very important feature that should be considered. Ideally there should not be any cracks or broken seals as this will contribute to the contamination of the purity levels of the oils.

Besides all this, the other important fact to consider is getting the best results through the method and choice of essential oils. Meaning some essential oil work better when used the correct way and the best results are assured if the recommended way is not taken for granted but adhered to carefully.

The method of inhalation is used to treat certain ailments like sinuses, headaches, colds, chest congestions and other similar conditions. This method is far more effective and quicker than taking oral or direct application on the skin.

Spraying a mixture of essential oils and distilled water is another method used to create a calming and relaxing atmosphere. This method has proved to be beneficial when treating anxiety, depression, stress and other pressurizing conditions.

Some conditions call for direct applications. However as most aromatherapy massage session are performed with direct skin contact, the concentration of the essential oils needs to be considered before commencing. Reason being that these essential oils could cause an allergic reaction to the individual.

CHAPTER 4- REASONS WHY YOU SHOULD CONSIDER AROMATHERAPY

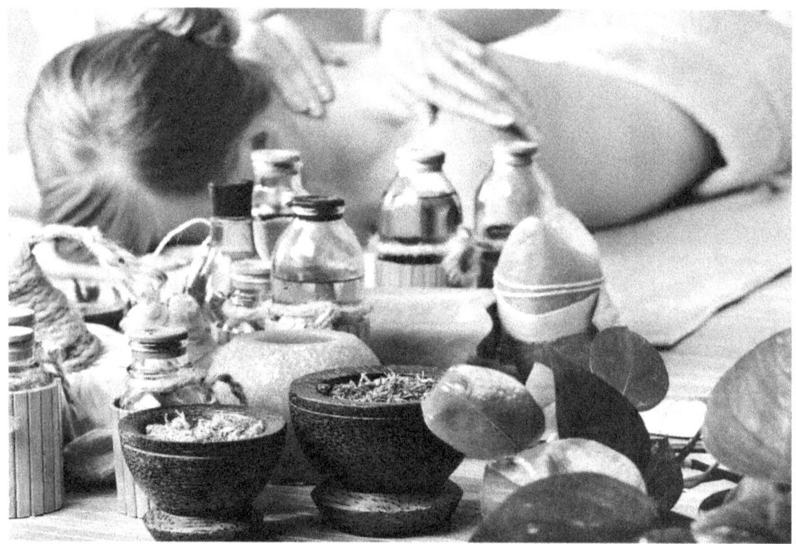

Commonly thought of as essential oils just for relaxing, therapeutic massage sessions, aromatherapy is fast gaining inroads into other areas. Some of which are forays into treating ailments and some medical conditions that have previous success rates from using aromatherapy methods.

For years some cultures have used aromatherapy to treat wound and scars effectively. Using essential oils that contain the Helichrysum ingredient has been proven to be beneficial when repairing damaged skin conditions.

Its strong anti-inflammatory and concentration of regenerative diketones is what makes it a highly regarded compound in addressing damaged skin problems. The pleasing earthy aroma it emits is also therapeutic.

Other essential oils that are also known for their healing properties for skin conditions are lavender, sage and rosemary. Sage is particularly effective in healing old scars and stretch marks but should only be used is small amounts because of the Thujone content which can be toxic.

Using aromatherapy to treat wounds is also widely practiced. This is because of the antiseptic elements that certain essential oils contain. Tea tree essential oil is commonly used to treat wound until the wound is totally sealed, after which this oil is no longer needed.

Some aromatherapy treatments are also used when the desire for healthy, younger looking skin is sought. These essential oils are absorbed into the skin and in turn provide the skin with all the important nutrients needed for the healthy look and condition.

Aromatherapy is also used in other products besides skin care. Products such as bath salts, shower gels, shampoos, body lotions. This style of using aromatherapy is wonderful for creating the desired effects of sweet smelling and relaxing moods. Also aromatherapy in this form is mild and non-threatening as it is not in its purest form.

Aromatherapy can also assist in relieving impatience and irritability. Essential oils like lavender can have calming effects on the mental turmoil state and works by encouraging the senses to slow down and simulates peace.

Approaching a medical condition by exploring the possibility of using aromatherapy as a solution is definitely worth the effort.

Aromatherapy ideally works when the psychological and physical aspects are addressed together. When the psychological and physical aspects are taken into account various contributing factors are studied carefully before any treatments are recommended.

The aroma therapist would have to consider factors like an individual's medical history, emotional condition, general health and lifestyle before putting forth any recommendations. This is a holistic style approach to treating a medical condition.

Some of the other more interesting conditions that are successfully explored using the aromatherapy method are backaches, irritable bowel syndrome, headaches and depression, to name a few. A good percentage of these medical ailments can be due to stress. Thus by using methods to understand and locate the individual's stress causing source, the aroma therapist will be able to alleviate the medical condition in a more efficient manner. In some extreme cases, claims of total recovery have been documented.

Treating skin problems is another avenue where aromatherapy has been successfully used. Conditions such as dermatitis, acne, eczema, psoriasis, cellulite, varicose veins and stretch marks are just some of the conditions where the use of essential oils has either arrested the condition or eradicated it completely.

Some patients have used aromatherapy to combat depression, hysteria, lack of concentration and panic attacks. Having tried other medically accepted methods which sometimes have undesirable side effects, aromatherapy has become a welcome solution. Treating burns, bruises and sprains using aromatherapy essential oils to achieve surprisingly quick and effective results are also another option worth exploring.

Other areas where the use of aromatherapy is being successfully explored are asthma, bronchitis, flu, and muscular aches and pains. When making the choice to use aromatherapy as a possible treatment for any given condition, it is important to ensure that only a qualified aromatherapy practitioner is consulted and that all the essential oils used are of the highest quality.

Chapter 5- The Healing Power of Aromatherapy

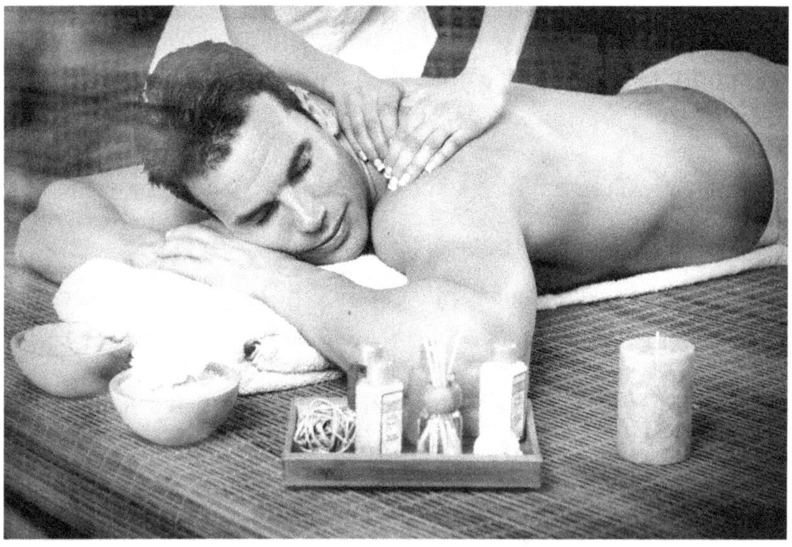

The popular belief that most illnesses and diseases are somehow linked to stress, anxiety and lack of proper daily nutrition has its merits.

Unfortunately some illnesses and diseases need to reach a critical stage before it becomes visible or is detected. To avoid all this, one is encouraged, though unrealistically, to keep all negative aspects in life under control or eliminate them altogether.

Aromatherapy can helpfully contribute to this end. Primarily known for its calming properties, aromatherapy methods advocate the use of various essential oils to soothe the mind and body. Besides this a long list of other conditions can be successfully addressed with the use of aromatherapy elements.

Below are just a few examples of the capabilities and merits of using aromatherapy:

- Acne – Lavender oil or tea tree oil to be applied directly onto the affected area. For milder cases, using a body bath lotion with these properties is recommended.

- Anemia – A concoction of tincture from the yellow dock root or an extract of dandelion leaf or even eating dandelion greens as a salad.

- Anxiety – Chamomile, California poppy, passion flower, lemon balm

- Asthma – Ginkgo biloba, mullein oil, and a Chinese herb called Shuan huang lian

- Bee sting – Urtica urens, cantharis, lavender and vegetable oil mixed

- Body odor – Alfalfa contains chlorophyll.

- Cold – Eucalyptus oil in boiling water and inhaled. Gargle with a mixture of tea tree oil

- Cholesterol – Chicory root, ginger

- Constipation – Aloe Vera juice, Ginger tea

- Hair loss – Saw palmetto, Arnica, Jojoba oil

- Headaches – Chamomile relaxes, Ginkgo biloba improves blood circulation

- Dandruff –Flaxseed oil, Primrose oil or Salmon oil. Rinsing hair in chaparral or thyme

- Diabetes – Huckleberry, tea made from most beans

- Diarrhea – Blackberry tea, wild oregano

- Eczema – Chickweed added to bath, Stinging nettle, Hazel ointment

- Indigestion – Gentian root for better digestion, Ginger, Peppermint

- Nausea and vomiting – Catnip leaves, Chamomile flowers

- Menopause – for skin use Geranium essential oil, Orange blossom water, Sandalwood essential oil

Fast gaining popularity as a new age fad, aromatherapy is only recently being taken seriously as a viable alternative treatment method to conventional medical remedies. For most ancient cultures this method of treatment has long been practiced with successful results.

Confusing the attributes that come with using the term aromatherapy is mainly caused by the commercial sector seeking to capitalize in this area. For many people aromatherapy is usually linked to some pleasing scent emitted from essential oils.

The effectiveness in the aromatherapy element is in the application and intent. Aromatherapy is meant to create a positive change physically, emotionally, mentally or spiritually which is supposed to directly impact the body condition of the person undergoing a session.

However when products are touted to use or contain essential oils for aromatherapy purposes without actually comprising of the much needed dosage, it is no longer considered aromatherapy.

Aromatherapy or commonly referred to as the practice of using essential oils for medicinal and therapeutic purposes covers many areas of healing properties. There are many essential oils used as remedies for various physical conditions and complaints. Essential oils are also believed to contain anti-viral, anti-fungal and antibacterial properties. There are also some essential oils that work well for various skin problems.

Chapter 6- Home Remedies Using Aromatherapy & Essential Oils

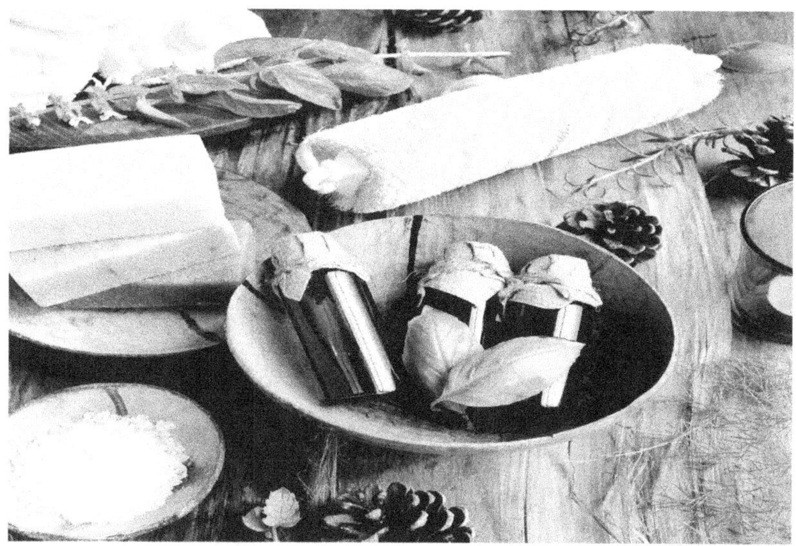

Natural Household Cleaners

The toxicity that household cleaners introduce into our homes goes far beyond the usual "harmful if swallowed" warning. In fact you don't need to consume household cleaners for them to poison you; your skin does a perfectly efficient job of doing that.

In fact, you can still be poisoned from the vapors of chemical cleaners and from being in contact with them.

Home Cleaner Recipes

Bathroom Air Freshener Spray

Fill a pump-spray bottle with 500ml of distilled water then add the following essential oils:

- 5 drops Cinnamon essential oil

- 5 drops Eucalyptus essential oil

- 5 drops Lemon essential oil

- 5 drops Sage essential oil

- 5 drops Thyme essential oil

- 10 drops Bergamot essential oil

- 10 drops Citronella essential oil

- 10 drops Lavender essential oil

- 10 drops Tea Tree essential oil

Shake this mixture well before each use. Spray every day to keep your bathroom smelling fresh and clean.

Lavender and Tea Tree Cleaner

- 1 t. borax

- 2 T. white vinegar

- 2 c. hot water

- 1/4 t. Lavender essential oil

- 3 drops Tea Tree essential oil

Mix all ingredients together and stir until dry ingredients dissolve. Pour into spray bottle for long-term storage and use. Spray as needed on any surface except glass. Scrub and rinse with a clean damp, cloth.

Disinfectant Spray

- 3 drops Cinnamon Leaf

- 5 drops Pine Needle

- 2 drops Frankincense

- 10 drops Bergamot

- 1/8 t. Sunshine Concentrate

- 30 ounces water

Combine essential oils with Sunshine Concentrate and water in a 32 oz. trigger spray bottle. Spray on and wipe surface dry. Disinfects countertops, stovetops and tile.

Microwave Cleaner

- 1/4 cup baking soda

- 1 teaspoon vinegar

- 6 drops lemon essential oil

Instructions: Mix ingredients to make a paste. Apply to interior of microwave with a sponge. Rinse and leave door open to dry for 15 minutes.

Wash the glass turntable by hand. This recipe will get rid of food odors.

Floor Cleaner

- 1/4 cup white vinegar to a bucket of water

- 10 drops lemon oil

- 4 drops oregano oil

Basic Wood Cleaning Formula

- 1/4 cup white distilled vinegar

- 1/4 cup water

- 1/2 teaspoon liquid castile soap

● 5 drops jojoba or olive oil

Combine the ingredients in a bowl. Saturate a sponge and squeeze out the excess. Wash surfaces of tired and dirty wood. The vinegar smell will dissipate soon. Dry with a soft cloth.

Creamy Soft Scrub

● 2 cups baking soda

● ½ cup liquid castile soap

● 4 teaspoons vegetable glycerin (acts as a preservative)

● 5 drops antibacterial essential oil such as lavender, tea tree, or rosemary.

For exceptionally tough jobs spray with vinegar first—full strength or diluted, scented—let sit and follow with scrub.

Sanitizing Deodorizer

● Add 1/2 (half) a cup of borax to 1 gallon (4 liters) of tepid warm water.

Can be used in place of your household cleaners and is just as effective as industrial strength brands without the potential harm to your health.

Tea Tree Oil Disinfectant

● 10 drops of tea tree oil (found at your local health shop)

● 10 drops of emulsifier

● 1 cup of water.

Add all of the ingredients together and mix thoroughly before use.

This recipe is almost identical to the cinnamon disinfectant recipe just substitute the cinnamon essential oil with tea tree essential oil.

These are cost effective; they last and are friendlier to your health and the health of the environment.

Natural Hair Care Treatments

Your hair is your crowning glory it's just a pity that what we put into it can leave it dry and dull and even brittle.

Here are some effective hair remedies that will infuse some much needed bounce and shine back into dull and lifeless hair.

For Greasy Hair

For your natural alternative to conditioner add 11 drops of rosemary and lavender to 25 ml of sunflower seed oil, add liberally and massage into the scalp. Bundle the hair up in a towel and leave in for 30 minutes. Before rinsing, apply your shampoo to help remove the oily conditioner treatment.

Dry Hair

Add 3 drops each of lavender and chamomile to every 5 ml of your pH balanced shampoo.

We're going to put a unique spin on our granny's old classic and add some extras to make it more sumptuous and smell less, castor oil-like.

Add 11 drop of chamomile and lavender with 25 ml of castor oil OR extra virgin olive oil, apply generously and gently massage throughout the hair, paying special attention the length of the hair shaft and the tips where hair is at its driest and most vulnerable.

Wrap the hair in a towel and leave for 30 minutes, for deep treatment, leave in for an hour.

Add in shampoo after leaving in for 30 minutes and work into lather before rinsing clear.

Wash the hair every 3 days to maintain the natural oils and to keep the frizz at bay.

Dandruff

Here are a couple of simple, yet effective treatments to help alleviate the symptoms of dandruff.

For a deep treatment add 20 drops of tea tree oil and 6 drops of lemongrass oil to 50 ml of coconut oil. Massage thoroughly paying special attention to the scalp area. Leave in for at least 30 to 40 minutes.

Before rinsing add 5 drops of tea tree oil to every 5 drops of pH balanced shampoo. Work into lather and rinse thoroughly until water runs clear.

Do this once a week.

During washes throughout the week, simply massage 4 to 5 drops of tea tree oil throughout the scalp and leave it in.

You should see a noticeable reduction in the amount of dandruff within two to three weeks.

Natural Cosmetics

Here are a few great homemade, organic recipes to make your own cosmetic creations from.

Beetroot Red Lipstick

That's right instead of crushing and adding iron to give your lipstick pigment, we're going to use something that isn't toxic and that you can eat any day of the week.

Add 1 tablespoon of grated beeswax from your local health store to 2 tablespoons of olive oil. Place in a microwavable glass dish and microwave on high for 2 minutes.

Then add 1 teaspoon of beet juice to the oily mixture. Mix thoroughly. Depending upon your taste, you can add more beet juice if you want a deeper, richer red color.

After mixing, let the mixture cool until it reaches room temperature then transfer the mixture to a small plastic container, apply using your finger or use a lipstick application brush and there you have it, non toxic, completely organic, lead free lipstick.

You have the flexibility to create different colors and tones by simply controlling the amount of beet juice that you add. Little beet juice gives a pink coloration. More beet juice gives the overall lipstick color a deep, rich red color.

Foundation/Concealer

First off we need to create our foundation/concealer mixture because it will also double up as the basis for our eye shadow.

Combine together an equal mixture of the following, 3 tablespoons of potato starch and 3 tablespoons of corn starch. If the mixture is lumpy, grind with the back of your tablespoon until fine.

To add some natural warm tones to your concealer, take 1 tablespoon of your foundation/concealer mixture that you just created and add a sprinkling of cinnamon until you get the desired tone for your skin color. Cinnamon is great for the skin, has healing properties and gives a beautiful natural scent without the use of harsh chemicals.

Eye Shadow

Combine 3 tablespoons of cocoa powder, any kind will do with 2 pinches of your home made concealer. By combining cocoa with your concealer mixture not only do you have color but your pre-made concealer mixture gives the eye shadow adhesion properties. The cocoa gives a natural looking warm tone to the eye shadow, if you want to add a little color you can purchase dry powder food coloring from your local cake shop. It's natural and its pigmentation is derived from plant extracts so you know it's beneficial to the skin.

Add the colored powder to your eye shadow mixture until you get the level of color desired. This is where you can depart from your standard nude warm tones and branch out into your blues, greens and purples.

Blush and Lip Gloss

To make the basis of your lip gloss add 2 tablespoons of sunflower oil to 1 tablespoon of beeswax beads, again you should be able to source any of these ingredients from your local health shop.

Place in a small cooking pot and heat until both have melted and combined together.

Add in a little pinch of beet powder for coloring, the more beet powder the darker and richer the color. Control the amount you put in until you get the desired color. If you want to save time, make 5 of these mixtures and add from a pinch in the first mixture and add a little more to the second batch until by the time you reach the final batch you've added a teaspoon.

Aromatherapy Remedies for Health and Wellbeing

Cracked skin

Cracked skin usually indicates a deficiency in vitamin's B2 and B6, thankfully you can infuse these vitamins naturally back into your body with diet. Believe it or not, liver is actually is a great source high in vitamin B. If liver's not your thing and you can't stand the taste then you can substitute it with wheat germ and even brewer's yeast. You shouldn't have any problems sourcing this from your local health shop.

Now that you're replacing the vitamins your body needs, you want to give your cracked skin some relief, wheat germ oil is ideal for this or alternatively, if you've got it in your kitchen pantry snap up a bottle Extra Virgin Olive Oil, anything that can act as a natural lubricant to re-infuse some that lost moisture will work well. The oil acts as a protective barrier to prevent further moisture loss and allow healing to take place.

A good bottle of EVOO works wonders and keeps skin supple, hydrated and reduces wrinkles.

Remember, during times of extreme cold to moisturize paying special attention to the neglected areas such as the hands and feet.

Warts

This is easy to do, but first you need to weaken the rough, fleshy wart exterior which protects these seeds. To break down the warty protective skin layer you need to soften it with tea tree oil by applying a few drops to the area 3 times daily for the next 30 days.

This callously exterior layer should soften and easily pull away enough for you to remove the seeds to prevent further growth and spreading.

Once you can see the black pepper dot seeds underneath the upper wart skin layer, sterilize a needle with antiseptic and gently dig out the seeds making sure to carefully dispose of them into a tissue.

Another connection scientists have made is that Vitamin E suppresses wart formation. Source out at your local health shop moisturizing creams containing vitamin E, this should give you a nice protective layer against those nasty little wart viruses.

Psoriasis

A great treatment for psoriasis is internal. By taking 6 doses of 500mg of Evening Primose Oil on a daily basis, 60% of people noticed a marked reduction in their symptoms.

A topical treatment you can use to give relief is to mix 5 teaspoons of cider vinegar with 3 fluid ounces of lavender water, 10 drops of lavender, cajeput and tea tree oil. Once combined, shake the mixture well and massage gently into your scalp 5 times per week.

Cold sores

Just dab a little tea tree oil onto the affected with a q-tip (cotton bud) and dispose of it in the trash. Remember that cold sores are a contagious virus of the Herpes family. By not disposing carefully of your q-tips or washing your hands thoroughly can potentially spread it to other parts of your body.

Repeat your tea tree oil treatment twice a day until the tingling sensation has disappeared and when the cold sore fails to develop.

So next time you get that tingling sensation, whip out your trusty tea tree oil.

To stop cold sores from appearing, boost your immune system by taking vitamin supplements. Vitamin C can either be introduced naturally through diet, kiwifruit especially of the golden variety are a fantastic source of vitamin C and contain up to 3 times that of your average Joe orange, weight to weight.

That's right; your regular sized orange only packs around 70 mg of vitamin C compared with 85 mg for one small golden kiwi. That means that you can eat just 2 golden kiwis to get your daily recommended dose of vitamin C a day.

Burns

Burns fall into 3 categories of severity.

Superficial: This involves some swelling and redness to the affected area.

Intermediate: Usually involves swelling the affected area accompanied by blistering of the skin.

Deep: Involves charring to the affected area often followed by a numbing feeling indicating tissue damage.

For burns in general, dose up on your garlic intake. Garlic is packed with healing properties. You can incorporate garlic naturally into your diet or if you're not keen on the taste, invest in some tasteless, odorless garlic capsules from your handy local health shop; it still packs a vitamin punch minus the garlic breath.

Treatment:

The first thing you should always do following a burn is to hold the affected area under a cold tap of running water for at least 15 minutes or more if need be. Apply tea tree oil to the affected area 3 times a day until the skin has fully healed.

For larger burn areas, apply a compress containing ice for 20 to 30 minutes or as long as need be.

Create a special mixture by combining 9 drops of lavender and 9 drops of German chamomile oil in 50 ml of distilled water. Combine the ingredients by shaking well and apply to the burn area. Continue to use until fully healed.

Essential oils are effective in the treatment of minor burns especially tea tree and lavender oils. They not only sooth the burned area but also help promote healing and prevent scarring. So effective are these oils that their use is being deployed more and more in hospitals for the treatment of burns.

Cuts

When it comes to rapid healing, vitamin C is highly effective accompanied with plenty of rest enabling the body to properly repair itself.

Eat foods loaded with vitamin C; a great source as mentioned previously is that of the golden kiwifruit. For its weight it packs a vitamin punch compared to its bigger, bulky fruity counterparts. That means that you can get more of your recommended daily intake from its snack sized portions.

Again, garlic is the "go to" healing elixir which helps boost the body's natural immune defenses and reduce infection.

When it comes to minor cuts and abrasions, as with burns, lavender is excellent because of its healing properties. In fact when applied to an affected area, lavender didn't sting to the touch as iodine does. Lavender promotes healing by stimulating a supply of blood to the damaged area. Not only does lavender help heal but it also prevents scarring.

Tea tree oil is another great natural antiseptic which draws infection from wounds and with its germicidal properties left affected areas clean and infection free unlike most commercial, chemically synthesized antiseptics which kills the bacteria and damages the tissue in the process.

Clean the affected wound area with water and apply 3 to 4 drops of lavender or tea tree oils. Apply a plaster taking the care to air the wound several times a day so that it doesn't become a breeding ground for bacteria. Apply the lavender or tea tree oil 3 times a day until healed.

For larger wound areas cover with gauze that has been dipped in tea tree or lavender oil. Add a few drops of yarrow or myrrh to the gauze, this will help promote healing.

Excessive Perspiration

Here's an effective way to treat perspiration without affecting your health.

First off, one of the simplest things that people tend to overlook is your internal health and by doing something as simple as drinking more water, you can dilute the amount of ammonia in your system that comes from a diet high in protein. You'll find doing this will reduce the strength in urine odor.

Wash your body regularly to remove the bacteria responsible for transforming your innocent perspiration into stench lactic acid. Use natural organic soaps containing tea tree oil which acts as a natural bactericide.

For the Feet

Add 5 drops of lavender and tea tree oil along with 1 tablespoon of cider vinegar to a bowl of warm water. Soak your feet each evening for at least 5 minutes. If you want extra soothing for tired aching feet add a few drops of lemon oil to the mix.

Natural Deodorant

Add 3 drops to of tea tree oil to witch hazel and rub liberally into the soles of the feet. It's also a great use as natural deodorant for the under arms too.

Lice

Between combing on a daily basis to remove the eggs, treat your hair by using a mixture of 1 to 3% of tea tree oil or lavender to a pH balanced shampoo from your local health shop. Massage thoroughly into the scalp and leave for 15 minutes before adding a few drops of lavender oil, lathering and rinsing completely.

You must continue this treatment until no more eggs are lodged in the lice comb and until you see no more evidence of lice still lingering.

Muscular Pain

Muscular pain can also be from a diet lacking in vitamin E. When you don't have enough vitamin E in your diet you experience tissue and muscular degeneration of which the symptoms are pain. By adding prime Rose oil supplement into your diet can greatly alleviate the symptoms of pain caused by this deficiency.

To relieve muscle aches massage is very effective especially with the right essential oils to promote pain relief.

You can create your own massage oil by using 10 drops of lavender, rosemary and marjoram oils to 50 ml of carrier oil. Apply to the affected area and massage until the oil is thoroughly worked into the muscle. This treatment is best suited after a warm shower or after application of a heat pack to loosen the aching muscle.

Another great remedy is to add 10 drops of chamomile to a hot bath and soak for 30 minutes to relieve aching muscles.

Cramp

To minimize the pain and frequency of cramps you need to look at your diet. Often cramps can be triggered by a lack of sodium (salt) in the diet. Garlic supplements are great for replenishing what you lack as are zinc and calcium supplements.

To treat muscular spasms of the extremities, namely the calf muscles and the hamstrings, create massage oil by adding 4 drops of marjoram, lavender and rosemary oils to 3 drops of ginger oil in 25 ml of cream.

To prevent the likelihood of cramping after extreme physical activity mix 10 drops of lavender, marjoram and rosemary oils with 45 ml of carrier oil (vegetable). Warm up the muscles with a warm shower or bath and apply the massage mixture to the affected area taking special care to thoroughly massage into the muscles until evaporated.

Hemorrhoids

Try to up your daily intake of fiber. A diet high in bran, cereals, fruits and vegetables enable the ease of removal of waste from your body, as does drinking plenty of fluids every day. Garlic and vitamin E supplements are also recommended.

To relieve yourself of the painful symptoms create yourself a soothing ointment by adding 5 drops of yarrow and 5 drops of germanium oil in 25 ml of calendula gel. Apply to the affected area 3 to 4 times per day or as necessary.

Another great way to gain relief is to add to 10 drops of rose oil to a bath of warm water and soak for 30 minutes.

Varicose Veins

Garlic supplements can help to heal within and just as beneficial, a diet high in fiber and vitamins E and C can also help to minimize the development of varicose veins as well as reduce the appearance of current ones.

To give relief to varicose and to help in the reduction of inflammation apply a cold compress to the affected area. To add even more relief, ensure that the compress is doused in witch hazel. This helps to sooth tired, aching legs.

Always remember to avoid taking hot baths, opt for warm, tepid ones. Hot baths only exacerbates the inflammation of the vein walls and causes them to ache even more.

The next time you take your warm, not hot bath try adding in 10 drops of juniper oil to improve circulation.

Constipation

It's important to expel your bowels of this harmful waste material to avoid building up toxicity in your body.

Ensure that you drink 2 glasses of warm, spring water before eating anything. This wakes up your digestive system in preparation for food. It also is a great way to clean out those kidneys following your 8 hours of sleep.

Try incorporating more vitamin B into your regular diet. Diets deficient in vitamin B can be linked to poor digestion and constipation. Try drinking senna or ginger tea at least once a day to help with constipation.

Here are a couple of natural remedies that can help alleviate the symptoms of constipation:

Apply directly to your abdominal area 4 drops of peppermint with 4 drops of ginger to 25 ml of almond oil, or the base oil of your choice and rub in circles. Do this 2 to 3 times a day.

To help relieve discomfort, use a flannel as a warm compress and add to the flannel 3 drops of peppermint and rosemary. Place on your abdomen for 30 minutes until pain begins to subside.

Another effective method of pain relief is to add 10 drops of peppermint oil to a warm bath, soak for at least 30 minutes. Do this as regularly as you need to.

Diarrhea

If your diarrhea isn't severe, just replenish your fluids and try these remedies.

If yours is derived from a bacterial infection, boost your immunity by taking garlic supplements. Drink plenty of fluids to replenish the fluids you've lost. The next time you take a drink of water, add a little salt to it to replace the salt you would have lost through excretion.

This is particularly effective for diarrhea as a result of stress, add to a warm bath 3 drops of ginger oil and 3 drops of lavender oil and soak for at least 30 minutes to relieve stress and tension.

If you're unwell from bacterial infection and have a fever, add 3 drops of peppermint oil and 3 drops of lavender oil to cool bath.

Toothache

If you've developed an abyss, garlic is great to help reduce the source of infection, reduce swelling and pain. Vitamin C will also encourage healing.

Before you get to your dentist there are things that you can personally do to help relieve the pain of a toothache.

Cloves are fantastic in the treatment of pain, add 2 drops of clove oil to a q-tip or cotton bud and apply to the affected tooth.

Using reflexology can also help to dull toothache pain. By massaging the area between thumb and forefinger or by rubbing a cube of ice in this area in circular motions can also help to dampen the pain.

To help fight infection, add 6 drops of tea tree oil to a 250 ml glass of tepid, warm water. Stir the mixture thoroughly. Swish around in your mouth paying special attention to the affected area. Do these twice a day directly after tooth brushing.

Another great pain relief method especially for aching pain and swelling is to create a special massage oil using 2 drops of peppermint oil mixed with 2 drops of lavender oil and add to 15 ml of olive oil which is your carrier oil. In a circular motion using your index and middle fingers, gently work the mixture into your cheek for 10 to 15 minutes or until pain begins to subside.

Colds

To keep your body as phlegm free as possible try to eat more fruits and vegetables in particular those rich in vitamin C such as golden kiwifruit, guavas, oranges and lemons.

Here are a few of my favorite cold remedies that you can put to work for you:

For a congested chest, make your own home made natural chest rub. Mix 5 drops of peppermint, thyme and ginger to 25 ml of almond carrier oil and massage into the chest and back until oil dries. Do this 2 to 3 times per day until chest clears.

For a stuffy head and sinuses, add to a boiling bowl of hot water, 6 drops of eucalyptus oil with 6 drops of tea tree oil. Place a towel over the head and inhale the vapor for 10 minutes. Ensure that your eyes are closed and that your face doesn't touch the surface of the water. Remember this is extremely hot water and can scold if not done carefully.

For sore throats, place 5 tablespoons of sea salt in a glass of tepid warm water and gargle and spit out. Repeat until all of the water is gone.

Give relief to tired achy and painful joints, by adding 10 drops of lavender and tea tree oil to hot bath and soak for at least 30 minutes. A hot bath eases the pain of painful joints and increases mobility while encouraging more peaceful, restful sleep.

Coughs

To alleviate coughing during times of chest infection use 5 drops of lavender oil and 5 drops ginger oil to 25 ml of carrier oil such as almond oil. Rub in circular motions into the chest, back and throat area (external use only). These essential oils act as expectorants and help to loosen and remove the mucus from your system.

A hot steam inhalation will give rapid relief to a dry, hacking cough. Add 3 drops of tea tree oil to 3 drops of sandalwood to a bowl of hot water. Cover your head with a towel and inhale the steam for 10 minutes. Repeat once in the morning and once at night.

Hay Fever

By cutting back on the amount of dairy you consume can alleviate hay fever symptoms. By also boosting your immune system with plenty of vitamin C and garlic and getting plenty of rest you can reduce the severity of hay fever symptoms normally experienced.

Try infusing your diet with immunity strengthening Manuka honey. Its healing properties can help better prepare your immune system when hay fever strikes.

To help clear out your nasal passages and to relieve head tension try adding 3 drops of lavender oil to 3 drops of rose oil to a tissue or a handkerchief and inhale. Once the mixture has evaporated and lost its potency, add another 3 drops of each again to replenish.

For relief of weeping, swollen and inflamed eyes, try placing a cucumber in the refrigerator for a couple of hours. Slice the cucumber into 1/2 inch pieces and place over each eye for 10 minutes for soothing eye relief.

Another great remedy is to add a teaspoon of rose water (not rose oil) into a cold, damp wash cloth and place over the eyes while closed. Leave on for 10 minutes. You can repeat this over again for as long as you need relief.

To reduce the frequency of coughing and sneezing and to relieve painful aftermath, combine 5 drops of lavender with 5 drops of rose oil and add to 25 ml of carrier oil. When applying and massaging, pay special attention to the neck and chest and rib area.

ABOUT THE AUTHOR

Margaret J. Bilkins became interested in healthy and natural remedies after giving birth to her beautiful twins. It made her much more concerned about creating a healthy lifestyle for her family. Through research and experimentation, Margaret has discovered some amazing recipes to help to improve overall health. Her finger tip guides, books and journals cover such topics as cleansing, aromatherapy and skin care recipes. She has worked hard to make available to help everyone get the vital information needed to maintain health in their busy lives.